CANDIDA
CAN
BE
BEATEN

How the 'innocuous' thrush can become the 'insidious' chronic mucocutaneous candidiasis and how it can be beaten.

Written by Richard Turner, B.Pharm., M.P.S.
Elizabeth Simonsen Registered Dietitian.

CANDIDA CAN BE BEATEN
How the 'innocuous' thrush can become the insidious' chronic mucocutaneous candidiasis and how it can be beaten.

Copyright © 1985 by Richard Turner and Elizabeth Simonsen
Reprinted 1986

Printed by The Dominion Press-Hedges and Bell, Maryborough, 3465

National Library of Australia
Cataloguing-in-Publication data

Turner, Richard, 1945-
    Candida can be beaten

    Includes index
    ISBN 0 9589510 0 4.

    1. Candidiasis. 2. Thrush (Mouth disease). 3. Candidiasis —
    Diet therapy. I. Simonsen, Elizabeth. II. Title.

616.9'69

Oidium Books, P.O. Box 191, CORIO, Vic. 3214, Australia

CANDIDA
CAN
BE
BEATEN

Richard Turner
Elizabeth Simonsen

Oidium Books,
P.O. Box 191,
CORIO, Vic., 3214
Australia

CONTENTS

CHAPTER 1

PROFILE ON
CANDIDA
ALBICANS

It was over 2,000 years ago that Hippocrates, the father of modern medicine, first described in his writings, a condition of the mouth and the vagina which was known as "thrush". But it was not until the 1850s, after Louis Pasteur developed the "germ theory" of disease, that the cause of the disease was identified as an infection of the skin or of the lining of the vagina or mouth by a microscopic organism known as Candida albicans, (sometimes known as Monilia albicans.)

Candida albicans is a type of yeast (not unlike baker's yeast) which is one particular sub group of the family of fungi or moulds. Fungi are quite familiar to us as mushrooms and as the "fur" which grows on spoiling bread or fruit. Yeasts, too, are familiar to us as an ingredient necessary to make the dough rise in the baking of bread, or in the brewing industry in the fermentation process to produce alcoholic drinks. Yeasts of various types are very widespread in our environment, occurring naturally in the soil and on the surfaces of almost all living organisms as part of the delicate eco-system of a myriad of microscopic living beings all existing in a sort of "love-hate" relationship with each other. Each one tolerates the other as long as the eco-system remains in balance and no one part of that system becomes dominant over any one of the other parts.

Moulds spread and reproduce by releasing into the atmosphere millions of spores, a sort of seed, yet so tiny as to float around in the air and eventually settle on a surface giving that surface the appearance of being dusty. If conditions are favourable, the spore will then grow into another mould "plant".

We all have, living on our skin surfaces, our own particular blend of yeast and other micro-organisms which live in harmony with each other and with their host. The linings of the human body (mucous membranes) can also be host to a cocktail of various micro-organisms without causing the least discomfort or disease. Candida albicans occurs normally on the skin and vagina and on the mucous membrane linings of the intestine and upper respiratory tract without causing any untoward reactions. But, as with any eco-system, when the natural balance is disturbed, then the resulting effects may be more widespread than anticipated.

A disturbance of the normal level of Candida is evidenced by symptoms of a "flare-up" of infection, as the discharge and itching of vulvo-vaginitis (vaginal thrush), the white coated tongue of oral thrush, as oesophagitis (heartburn) and the abdominal discomfort, distension, constipation, diarrhoea and rectal itching that goes with yeast infection of the bowel.

Dr Orion Truss, in his book "The Missing Diagnosis" suggests that the widespread use of antibiotics, combined with the use of birth control pills and of immunosuppressant (cortisone type) drugs, coupled with a prolonged high, simple carbohydrate diet (fast food type) has caused a dramatic change in that delicate relationship which we have with the micro-organisms which live on our skin and mucous membranes. This causes such a disturbance to the fragile eco-system as to be a major cause of the disease which is outwardly benign, yet can be so debilitating, that of CHRONIC CANDIDIASIS.

CHAPTER 2

IMMUNE REACTIONS TO FOODS, INHALANTS, CHEMICALS AND CANDIDA TOXINS

Allergies to substances in our environment are not new – Hippocrates wrote about "allergic reactions" and since Roman times, Lucretius has been credited with observing that "one man's meat is another man's poison". However, the number and frequency of allergic reactions seems to be increasing for a variety of reasons.

Under normal circumstances, our body's immune system will be activated when the body is invaded by any matter which the immune system can identify as being foreign to the individual. The foreign matter may be pollen, bacteria, viruses, chemical pollutants in the air, chemicals applied to the skin, chemicals ingested with food (which may be of synthetic or natural origin) or even improperly digested food fragments.

Following invasion of the body by foreign matter (usually protein) a competent immune system will isolate and destroy the foreign material. If, for any reason, the immune system fails to completely detoxify all foreign material entering the body, then that material can be circulated to all parts of the body where it can bring about its toxic reaction, which may be congestion of the sinuses, precipitation of an asthma attack, behavior modification, headache or any one or many of a whole host of symptoms affecting any part of the body. We are all familiar with the way some people suffer hay fever during the grass pollen season, or the way some people get hives after eating strawberries or oranges. In the same way, any foreign material is capable of causing an allergic reaction in an individual whose immune system is in any way compromised.

Many factors influence how well the immune system is able to cope with a quantity of foreign material (allergenic load):

1. adequate nutrition,
2. stress,
3. allergenic load.

Like all body systems, the immune system needs an adequate supply of vitamins and minerals, especially vitamins A, B6, and C and zinc in the correct proportions. The chemical changes in the body brought about by any type of stress actually suppress the immune system. And stress can be of physical (infection or injury) or emotional origin. These factors are so important as to warrant separate chapters within this book.

One's allergenic load is the quantity of foreign matter which is allowed to invade the body. Substances which contribute to the allergenic load include: chemical pollutants inhaled with the air we breathe, dust, pollen, bacteria or mould spores inhaled, chemicals either as pollutants or additives to the food we eat, naturally occurring contaminants of food such as natural poisons, bacteria, yeast or viruses or products of their breakdown. Many chemical pollutants increase the occurrence of abnormal cells in the body and it is the responsibility of the immune system to destroy those too.

Like all living matter, the yeast cell is a very complex group of chemicals which are released when the yeast cells die or are digested. These chemicals may be absorbed from the gut into the bloodstream and circulated throughout the body. Many of these chemicals have been positively identified as being toxic to the brain which explains how a heavy load of yeast products can be the cause of behavioral disturbances. Normally, these chemicals would not be absorbed from the gut, but Candida has the ability to transform itself to a mycelial form in the gut and burrow into the intestinal wall which irritates the gut lining to the extent that it permits substances to cross into the bloodstream which the gut lining would normally exclude.

It is easy to see how a poor diet can compromise the immune system by:

1. providing an inadequate supply of vitamins and minerals,
2. encouraging a Candida flare-up and thus adding to the allergenic load.

CHAPTER 3

RISK FACTORS AND DIAGNOSIS OF CHRONIC CANDIDIASIS

It is extrememly important to realise that many of the symptoms described here can be the manifestation of many disorders other than those related to Candida, and that it is important to have a thorough examination by your physician to rule out that possibility before making the assumption that the cause is Candida.

As Candida is present in almost everyone, healthy or ill, it is practically impossible to devise a laboratory test that will positively identify Candida as the causative agent. Some rather expensive blood tests can point to the possibility only, that Candida is the cause, so diagnosis relies on the presence of symptoms and risk factors which appear in a thorough medical history. Following the history, an accurate diagnosis can be confirmed by an improvement in the conditon as a result of instituting anti-Candida treatment.

Chronic Candidiasis is more likely to be the diagnosis if the history shows:

Repeated or prolonged courses of BROAD SPECTRUM ANTIBIOTICS, especially for repeated or recurrent sinus or ear infections, or bronchitis or acne. Antibiotics suppress the micro-organisms in the intestine which live in competition with yeasts and thus allow the yeast colonies to "flare up".

Courses of CORTISONE, PREDNISOLONE OR OTHER CORTICOSTEROIDS for skin rashes, asthma or arthritis. These drugs suppress the body's own natural immune system and again allow a "flare up" of yeasts anywhere in the body.

MULTIPLE PREGNANCIES with or without courses of BIRTH CONTROL PILLS or other hormone preparations. These situations produce a level of hormones in the body which encourage yeast growth.

A prolonged HIGH CARBOHYDRATE DIET, especially of simple carbohydrates such as sugars and white flour preparations. Simple carbohydrates like these are the very foods on which yeast cells thrive and therefore encourage a proliferation of yeast cells in the intestine.

In the experience of Candida patients, almost all symptoms imaginable have occurred and have been relieved by successful anti-Candida treatment. But some symptoms seem to appear more frequently in patients' medical histories which tend to pinpoint Candida as the prime suspect:

Recurrent or chronic infections of the vagina or urinary system suggest a chronic Candida infection which can lead to other disorders of the sex organs such as fluid retention, endometriosis, period pain and cramps, irregular menstrual bleeding and an impairment or loss of sex drive.

Recurrent or chronic infections of the skin, especially around the finger and toe nails, recurrent "athlete's foot" infection, "jock itch" or psoriasis suggest a chronic yeast problem.

Depression, especially in women, associated with a continual tiredness and lethargy suggests a tired immune system. This may be associated with other vague nervous system symptoms such as inability to concentrate, poor memory, headache, pre-menstrual tension, explosive temper outbursts, inco-ordination, irritability, drowsiness, loss of self confidence, crying spells, loss of reasoning ability or inability to sleep.

Cravings for sweet and carbohydrate rich foods which provide a supply of food for the yeast colonies in the intestine or craving for yeast foods such as cheese, bread, yeast and malt extracts, and especially alcoholic beverages also suggest a yeast allergy.

Symptoms which are aggravated by tobacco smoke, car or diesel exhaust fumes, perfumes or other chemical odours.

Symptoms which are worse on damp, humid days or while in damp, mouldy places. At these times the mould level in the atmosphere is much higher and there are much more mould spores floating about.

Persistent digestive problems such as heartburn, indigestion, bloating and gas, abdominal distension and pain, constipation or diarrhoea or alternating bouts of both are all symptoms which suggest a "flare-up" of yeast colonisation of the gastro-intestinal tract.

Recurrent sore throats, nasal congestion or cough, point to Candida colonisation of the sinuses.

Other vague symptoms which have been reported include pain and swelling in the joints, pain or tightness in the chest, blurred vision or spots before the eyes, ringing in the ears, cold extremities, or just plain "feeling poorly".

CHAPTER 4

SYMPTOMS KNOWN TO HAVE BEEN ASSOCIATED WITH CHRONIC CANDIDIASIS

A definite diagnosis of Chronic Muco-cutaneaous Candidiasis is practically impossible. Only a series of vague symptoms shows the patient that everything is not well, but no end of medical examinations and pathology tests will confirm a definite disease.

The symptoms and conditions listed are known to have occurred with chronic Candidiasis, not always together, and not always severe, but all have been experienced by patients to some degree and all have been relieved by anti-Candida therapy. In medical circles, diseases are traditionally grouped according to the organ or system which is affected and we have tended to go off to the appropriate specialist to solve the problems associated to his particular specialty. However, Candida toxins affect all cells of all organs and systems thus causing all the symptoms listed below. They are grouped according to custom for convenience although the whole picture must be considered during diagnosis.

The symptoms known to have been experienced include:

CENTRAL NERVOUS SYSTEM (MENTAL) SYMPTOMS

Depression, especially in women and especially in the week preceding menstruation.

Loss of self confidence.

Agitation.

Explosive irritability.

Sudden crying spells.

Loss of memory.

Confusion.

Inability to concentrate.

Loss of reasoning ability.

Dizziness.

Insomnia.

Disturbances of smell, taste, sight or hearing.

Headaches.

Hyperactivity, especially in children.

Inappropriate drowsiness.

Numbness, tingling and muscle weakness.

GASTRO-INTESTINAL SYMPTOMS

Heartburn.

Indigestion.

Bloating and flatulence.

Abdominal pain.

Persistent diarrhoea or constipation or alternating bouts of both.

Coated tongue.

Perianal (around the anus) itching.

GENITO-URINARY SYMPTOMS

Fluid retention.

Menstrual bleeding irregularities.

Menstrual cramps.

Endometriosis.

Loss of libido.

Urgency or frequency of urination.

Bed-wetting,

MUSCULO-SKELETAL SYMPTOMS

Muscle aches and cramps.

Pain and swelling of the joints.

UPPER RESPIRATORY TRACT SYMPTOMS

Persistent nasal congestion or sinusitis.

Recurrent sore throats.

Chronic cough.

Chronic or recurrent bronchitis.

SKIN AND MUCOUS MEMBRANES

Chronic or recurring mouth ulcers.

Itchy scalp and dandruff

Red, scaly eyelids.

Recurrent fungous infections of the skin including the nails and "jock itch".

Athlete's foot or tinea infections.

Psoriasis.

ALLERGIC SYMPTOMS

Most of the symptoms described above are the result of an allergic reaction to the toxic yeast metabolites but symptoms may also be precipitated by exposure to other substances such as foods and chemicals.

CHAPTER 5

PRINCIPLES OF TREATMENT OF CHRONIC CANDIDIASIS

In previous chapters, we have seen how deceitful Candida can be, in the way that the disease slowly creeps up on the unsuspecting patient, and then lies hidden under a cloak of confusingly vague symptoms and feelings, giving a glimpse of itself here and there but refusing to allow a simple diagnosis of the insidious condition it causes.

Typical of Candida, neither will it allow us to wipe it out with a simple course of antibiotics, because it quickly re-establishes itself just like before — simply because the immune system is too exhausted to cope with a flare-up of Candida yeast infection. Treatment is therefore aimed at allowing the immune system to have a rest from the constant bombardment of yeast metabolites (toxic chemicals released when a yeast cell dies) which can be accomplished by a variety of measures. Yeast metabolites absorbed into the bloodstream can originate either from a die-off of yeast cells in the gut, or from yeast containing foods. Some very sensitive individuals can even absorb enough yeast metabolites through the lungs from yeast spores inhaled in the air they breathe.

Your practitioner will use a combination of one or more of the following treatment measures to control the Candida infection and allow re-establishment of a competent immune system.

A. SUPPRESS THE YEAST LIVING IN THE GUT
1. By taking a specific anti-yeast type of antibiotic.
2. By modification of the diet and lifestyle to starve the offending yeast and thereby supress its growth.
3. By avoidance of medications which promote yeast growth such as the contraceptive pill, antibiotics and cortisone.

B. REST AND STIMULATE THE IMMUNE SYSTEM
1. By avoidance of foods which contain yeast metabolites.
2. By identification and avoidance of chemicals and other foods to which you may be allergic.
3. By avoidance of exposure to yeast spores in the atmosphere.
4. By avoidance of drugs which suppress the immune system such as cortisone and other immuno-suppressant drugs.
5. By use of extracts of Candida albicans to stimulate the immune system.
6. By use of vitamin and mineral supplements to assist regeneration of the immune system.

SUPPRESSION OF THE YEAST WITH A SPECIFIC ANTI-CANDIDA ANTIBIOTIC

The most commonly used specific anti-yeast antibiotic is nystatin (Mycostatin or Nilstat) which is a highly purified substance derived from the bacteria: Streptomyces noursei. Nystatin is a bitter tasting pale yellow powder which is insoluble in water. It is available on prescription as capsules, tablets and mixture for internal use, as creams and ointments for use on the skin and as vaginal pessaries and creams for use in the vagina. Nystatin is the preferred drug because it is very poorly absorbed from the gut into the bloodstream so is safe to take even in large quantities with little likelihood of toxic side-effects.

Treatment is usually begun by taking one capsule (or tablet) four times a day (approximately every six hours as that is the period of time that Candida takes to flare-up). At the same time, it is best to treat any affected skin areas by use of an appropriate nystatin preparation for application to the skin, nails or vagina. Over a period of weeks, the oral nystatin may be gradually increased to sixteen capsules per day (four, four times daily) or less if symptoms are relieved at a lower dosage. The appropriate maintenance dosage is different for each individual and must be established after several weeks by slowly reducing the dose of nystatin until symptoms re-occur. The maintenance dose is the minimum required to control symptoms.

Nystatin is generally well tolerated by most people but may cause nausea in some individuals. Some individuals who are very sensitive may react to the non-active ingredients in the tablet or capsule and can tolerate only the pure powder stirred into water. It has a bitter taste, but is tolerable.

Commencement of a course of nystatin at low dosage levels is important if we are to avoid the after effects of "die-off". Whenever there is a severe infection of Candida in the gut, a large dose of nystatin would cause large numbers of Candida yeast cells to "die-off" which would result in the release of a much larger than normal quantity of yeast metabolites, which, when carried to other parts of the body in the bloodstream cause toxic reactions which are easily recognisable as uncomfortable symptoms. Sometimes, these reactions to the massive release of toxic metabolites can be quite severe but this can be avoided by gradually increasing the nystatin.

Other anti-yeast antibiotics which can be used are amphotericin (Fungilin) and ketoconazole (Nizoral). Both of these antibiotics tend to be absorbed into the bloodstream to a greater extent than is nystatin, and consequently are more likely to lead to toxic side effects—especially in individuals with impaired liver function. For that reason, amphotericin and ketoconazole are generally reserved for the more stubborn cases.

STARVATION OF THE YEAST BY DIET MODIFICATION

Yeasts thrive on highly processed carbohydrate like sugar and white flour. It therefore follows that the yeast flare-up can be prevented by modifying the diet so as to eliminate simple carbohydrates. This is such an important part of the treatment of chronic Candidiasis that it is the subject of most of the rest of this book.

AVOIDANCE OF YEAST PROMOTING MEDICATIONS

Flare-up of a Candida infection is encouraged by some prescribed medications, which, if avoided, can significantly reduce yeast growth. Antibiotics, especially broad spectrum antibiotics, upset the normal bacteria-yeast balance in the gut by suppressing the bacteria and allowing the yeast to flare-up. Certain hormone preparations, including the contraceptive pill, change the metabolic pattern in the body in a way which encourages yeast growth. Then there are the immunosuppressant or cortisone type drugs, which, as the name suggests, suppress or weaken the immune system. The weakened immune system is then less able to cope with the chronic Candida infection with the unavoidable result being a flare-up of the Candida infection.

A course of any of these drugs can encourage a temporary flare-up of a Candida infection but these drugs are often taken for years on end and also sometimes a combination of two, or even all three types of drugs are taken together and all are encouraging yeast growth. Avoidance of the yeast promoting medications is important in assisting to reduce the possibility of yeast flare-up.

RESTING OF THE IMMUNE SYSTEM BY AVOIDANCE OF YEAST FOODS

Whenever our bodies are tired or unwell, the best recovery follows a period of bed rest. However, we cannot put our immune system to bed for a rest, but we can help by reducing the workload. The immune system is a system of protection against any chemicals which it identifies as being foreign to our bodies. Any chemicals which the immune system identifies as being foreign are normally quickly detoxified or neutralized and excreted. The most common source of foreign chemicals is from improperly digested foodstuffs which may be absorbed from the gut, especially if the gut lining is damaged by a chronic Candida infection. One way of reducing the load on the immune mechanism is to reduce the amount of toxic chemicals in the gut. As yeast cells are a source of many troublesome toxic chemicals, reducing the amount of yeast in the diet will assist the immune system to rest and recuperate. Yeast foods include bread, cheese, wine and beer, which with many others listed in Chapter 7, are foods to be avoided.

IDENTIFICATION AND AVOIDANCE OF CHEMICALS AND OTHER ALLERGENS

There are thousands of chemicals, foreign to our bodies, polluting the atmosphere and elsewhere in the environment — especially in food. All of these chemicals, when absorbed into the bloodstream have to be detoxified by the immune system and all add to the allergenic load on the immune system.

The immune system can be relieved of much of this load by avoidance of exposure to chemical pollutants such as vehicle fumes, industrial pollutants, food crop sprays, preservatives, stabilizers, emulsifiers and all the other chemicals added to processed food.

Similarly, foods to which we are allergic, place an extra burden on the immune system. An allergenic reaction is brought about by some improperly digested protein being identified by the immune system as being foreign and requiring detoxification. Causes of food intolerances need to be identified and avoided in order to reduce the workload of the immune system.

Inhaled allergens (usually pollens) place an added burden on a weakened immune system and should be avoided if possible, although that may be rather difficult. Air filters or negative ion generators may help.

AVOIDANCE OF EXPOSURE TO YEAST SPORES

When mould cells mature, they release millions of microscopic spores into the atmosphere where they can be carried great distances by the wind. The spores are breathed in with the air and lodge in the nasal passages or breathing tubes by the normal air cleaning mechanisms, where they are carried along with the mucus which usually eventually ends up in the stomach and gut, where the spores may be digested or may lead to infection. Either way, they release yeast metabolites which require detoxification by the immune system. Avoidance of mouldy or musty areas and cleaning up mould in the bathroom can help to reduce the load on the immune system. Other mould avoidance measures are described in Chapter 11.

AVOIDANCE OF IMMUNOSUPPRESSANT DRUGS

The cortisone type drugs not only allow Candida infections to flare up, but, at the same time, actually suppress the immune system. This immunosuppressant action is beneficial when the immune system gets out of hand and starts to attack some of the body's normal chemicals. But when the aim is to regenerate an effective immune system, these types of drugs should be avoided if possible.

STIMULATION OF THE IMMUNE SYSTEM WITH CANDIDA EXTRACTS

"Allergy extracts" or "vaccines" consist of injectable products which contain ingredients to which the patient has become allergic. Candida albicans extract is derived from Candida albicans cells and bottled in such a way that it may be injected. This is used in carefully controlled doses designed to stimulate the body's normal chemicals. When the aim is to regenerate metabolites. The goal is to replace the normal allergic reaction with an immune response, so that symptoms no longer result on exposure to that allergen.

AIDING THE IMMUNE SYSTEM BY SUPPLEMENTATION WITH VITAMINS AND MINERALS

Many mal-digestion and mal-absorption problems can lead to poor absorption of some vitamins and minerals. At the same time, any detoxification exercise undertaken by the immune system involves the consumption of vitamins and minerals, especially vitamin C. Supplementation of vitamins and minerals is aimed at providing the immune system with all the raw materials necessary for it to do its job, and also to recover its normal functioning capacity. Vitamin supplementation is the subject of Chapter 10.

CHAPTER 6

BASIC DIETARY GUIDELINES

With or without the use of anti-Candida antibiotics, Candida is most unlikely to be beaten without a major modification of diet and lifestyle. Modifications to diet are aimed at restricting the allergenic load by restricting the amount of yeast products in the diet and also restricting the quantity of refined and simple carbohydrates on which the Candida thrives. A combination of these measures has been found to greatly improve the recovery rate in treatment of chronic Candidiasis. It is important to restrict the amount of carbohydrate (especially refined carbohydrate), but, at the same time provide the host with a better than adequate diet in order to assist recovery.

In planning any diet, it is important to follow the "Dietary Guidelines for Australians" as laid down by the Dietetics Association of Australia. An adequate diet is achieved by consuming a balanced combination of a variety of five basic

food groups:
1. CEREALS.
2. PROTEIN FOODS including meats, fish, eggs, beans and lentils.
3. MILK AND DAIRY PRODUCTS.
4. VEGETABLES AND FRUITS.
5. BUTTER, MARGARINE OR OILS.

Proper nutrition is provided by a combination of protein, fats, carbodydrate, vitamins and minerals. The five food groups mentioned above provide a combination of all these essentials in varying proportions. As an example, a cereal grain has a different combination of protein, fats, carbohydrate, vitamins and minerals from a serve of chicken with gravy. All five food groups (before processing) contain vitamins and minerals. Groups 1 to 4 contain carbohydrates of various types. Carbohydrate is an essential nutrient as it provides our immediate energy needs, or if not immediately required, is converted to fat stores in the body.

Carbohydrates are considered to be either simple (small molecule) or complex (large molecule). Complex carbohydrates in the diet are broken down by normal digestion (partly by saliva) into simple carbohydrates. As a general rule, the simpler the carbohydrate, the sweeter the taste. It is these simple carbohydrates on which the Candida yeast in the gut thrives. The most commonly occurring simple carbohydrate in the Western diet is cane sugar (sucrose) which is the highly purified and most factory prepared foods. Simple sugars do occur is used extensively as a sweetener in soft drinks, cakes, biscuits, jams and jellies, most packaged breakfast cereals, confectionery and most factory prepared foods. Simple sugars do not occur in unrefined foods like milk and fruit. These foods contain their own sugars which, with care, can be included in a restricted carbohydrate diet. Honey contains an especially high concentration of simple sugars and should be avoided where possible.

Complex carbohydrates or starches are more slowly digested in the intestine to simple sugars so are more slowly absorbed, but, at the same time, do not provide the large concentrations of simple sugars which encourage yeast growth. Foods rich in complex carbohydrates are also rich in fibre, which is another important part of the overall diet. Foods rich in complex carbohydrates include all grains, seeds, beans, peas, nuts and vegetables.

The following chart shows how the refining of food alters the nutrient value of that food:

	2 apples	1 cup apple puree	½ cup apple juice
Fibre Content	high	low (broken down)	nil
Kilojoule Content	high	high	high
Eating time	slow	fast	fastest
Carbohydrate Absorption Rate	slow	faster	very fast

DIET TO BEAT CANDIDA

The diet to beat Candida is basically: yeast free and low in carbohydrate.

Depending on the rate of recovery, it may be necessary to follow the diet specified by your practitioner for from 3 months to 3 years, although the strictness of the diet may also vary. As with all diets, it is advisable to plan ahead and ensure that appropriate ingredients are on hand to prepare a meal which is not in contravention of the diet.

Remember, yeast free and low in carbohydrate — plan for 10 to 12 average sized serves of medium carbohydrate dishes per day, spread evenly across all meals and include a good variety of other foods.

CHAPTER 7

FOODS
TO BE
AVOIDED

YEAST FOODS

Avoid, as much as possible, all foods whose preparation involves the use of yeast or yeast products such as:

Antibiotics derived from moulds such as pencillin, erythromycin and tetracycline and also meat from livestock which has been fed antibiotic supplemented feed (usually pork).

Beer, brandy, champagne, cider, gin, ginger beer, rum, vodka, whisky, wine and other fermented alcoholic beverages.

Breads and other yeast raised baked goods including rolls, coffee scrolls, Easter and other buns and some pastries.

Brewer's yeast (as a dietary supplement).

Cheeses, especially the hard, matured cheeses. Not including cottage cheese and cream cheese, sour cream and sour milk products.

Condiments such as chutney and tomato and soy sauce, and spices.

Dried and candied fruits including sultanas, raisins, muscatels, dates, apricots, prunes and figs.

Fruit juices commercially prepared including orange, apple and tomato. Canned or tinned fruits and vegetables (manufacturers are not always careful to avoid inclusion of any mouldy fruit)

Fruit or vegetables that are showing the least signs of bruising or mould.

Malt containing products such as malted drinks, Milo, sweets and many prepared breakfast cereals.

Melons, especially canteloupe.

Mushrooms, champignons and truffels (fungi).

Peanuts and pistachio nuts usually contain mould.

Pickled, smoked or otherwise processed meats and fish, including sausages, hot dogs, corned beef, pastrami and pickled fish such as herrings.

Tea, herb teas and coffee.

Vinegar (distilled from grain, apple, wine, rice or other sources) and vinegar containing foods such as mayonnaise, salad dressings, mustard, sauces (tomato, Worcestershire, barbecue), pickles, pickled vegetables, relishes, green olives and sauerkraut.

Vitamins of the B complex group (either alone or in multi-vitamin preparations) as they are often derived from yeast.

HIGH CARBOHYDRATE FOODS

The foods to be avoided in this category are those which contain simple sugars and simple starches which are very rapidly converted to sugar in the body. They are:

Honey and other natural sweeteners including molasses, maple syrup, raw sugar, golden syrup and brown sugar. Pastries, cakes, biscuits, pancakes, donuts, puddings, bread rolls, scones, pies, tarts, spaghetti and other pasta, thickened soups and sauces, pizza or any other food which contains refined (white) flour. That includes refined flour made from wheat, corn, rice, or any other source. Sugar and sugar containing foods. This includes most of the sweet pastries, cakes, biscuits, donuts, puddings, pies and tarts mentioned above, as well as jams, jellies, confectionery, canned fruits, cordials, soft drinks, icy poles and ice cream, fruit juice drinks and all other foods containing sugars. It is essential to read the ingredient lists on the labels of all processed foods as practically all processed foods contain sugar of some sort. Also, they may be listed by their proper names which include: sucrose, fructose, maltose, lactose, glucose, dextrose, mannitol, sorbitol, galactose or corn syrup.

All of these ingredients encourage yeast growth in the gut and are best avoided. A small amount of sweetener in a recipe which serves several people only provides a very small quantity for one service which may not be sufficient to cause problems. However, it is best to avoid them completely where possible. It probably sounds impossible at this stage, but please read on to Chapters 8 and 9 where there are lists of lots of foods which are wholesome, nutritious, and tasty, and which may be eaten with little restriction.

CHAPTER 8

ALLOWED FOODS

As a basic dietary guideline, your diet should consist of as wide a variety as possible of a well balanced combination of foods from each of the 5 food groups. This ideal may have to be compromised if food intolerances are present but should include some:

CEREALS which may include wholegrain products either home-made or obtained from a recognised safe source of: barley, buckwheat, corn (maize), millet, oats, rice, triticale or wheat.

PROTEIN FOODS which must be fresh, or if quick frozen, should be thawed and used immediately and can include:

Meats including beef, veal, lamb, mutton, pork and game meats.

Poultry including chicken, turkey, duck, goose and quail.

Fish of salt or freshwater origin as well as shellfish (oysters, mussels, scallops, etc.) crustaceans (crayfish, lobster, crab, prawns, shrimp etc.)

Eggs of chicken, duck or quail.

Nuts and seeds such as almonds (in shells) Brazil nuts, cashew, macadamia and pecan nuts and pumpkin, sesame and sunflower seeds.

Lentils or dried beans.

Sprouts of alfalfa and beans freshly prepared.

MILK AND DAIRY PRODUCTS including cow and goat milk, but not in excessive quantities due to its high lactose content. Some prepared milk products such as yoghurt, cottage and ricotta cheese and buttermilk are allowed and recipes are provided in Chapter 9.

VEGETABLES AND FRUITS. All fresh vegetables (except mushrooms and champignons) and frozen vegetables are allowed if used immediately and not re-frozen. Includes asparagus, beets, broccoli, Brussel sprouts, cabbage, carrots, cauliflower, celery, corn, cucumber, eggplant, green and red peppers, lettuce, onions, parsley, peas, beans and legumes, parsnip, potato, pumpkin, radish, squash, spinach, silver beet, tomato and zucchini.

Fruits tend to contain more simple sugars than vegetables so should not be consumed in excess. All are allowed (except grapes and canteloupe which have a lot of yeast naturally occurring on their skins) and include: apple, avocado, banana, all berries, cherries, grapefruit, kiwi fruit, lemon, mango, mandarine, nectarine, orange, peach, pear, paw paw, pineapple, plum, tangerine and apricot.

BUTTER, MARGARINE OR OILS are allowed but should not be consumed in excess of 4 to 8 teaspoonfuls per day.

Oils may be from any source material such as almond, apricot, corn, linseed, olive, corn, safflower, sesame or sunflower.

CHAPTER 9

RECIPES
AND SAMPLE
DIET PLANS

The last three Chapters have described the basic rules for the design of an anti-Candida diet — by the restriction of carbohydrate rich foods and by the avoidance of yeast based and refined carbohydrate foods. This Chapter will show how a tasty, nutritious diet can be enjoyed without going outside the guidelines.

Your practitioner will have decided what would be your optimum level of carbohydrate intake. Here is an easy way to keep track of your daily consumption of carbohydrate. Each recipe or diet plan idea has beside it, a symbol which indicates the approximate carbohydrate content per average sized serve.

N for negligible or no carbohydrate,
L for low carbohydrate, (equals half of one M serve)
M for medium carbohydrate.

Aim to consume only 10 to 12 average sized serves of M dishes per day.

The diet plans described here are samples only, to act as a starting point in a fairly dramatic change of lifestyle, and should be used as a basis for broadening the range of foods consumed on a regular basis.

BREAKFAST SUGGESTIONS

A serve of fresh fruit or freshly squeezed juice.
Cooked oatmeal, rye or millet flakes with yoghurt or milk.
Puffed wholegrain wheat or rice with yoghurt or milk.
Eggs, cooked any style.
Grilled lamb chop or steak with grilled tomato.
Potato pancakes.
Biscuits, damper, pancake or other bread substitute.
Butter or margarine.

LUNCH SUGGESTIONS

Home made vegetable soup.
Meat, fish, poultry, egg or cottage cheese.
Salad.
Biscuits, damper, pancake or other bread substitute.
Butter or margarine.
Fresh fruit.

MAIN MEAL SUGGESTIONS

Home made soup.
Meat, poultry or fish with potato, yellow and green vegetables.
Fresh fruit.
Yoghurt.

PACKED LUNCH SUGGESTIONS

Sandwich of bread substitute with butter or margarine and filled with chopped chicken, grated carrot and chopped celery moistened with a little yoghurt. For variety, use other allowed meats with alfalfa sprouts, shredded lettuce or watercress. Pack pieces of meat and salad vegetables with a separate sandwich of bread substitute and butter or margarine.

Fresh fruit.

Yoghurt.

AFTER SCHOOL SNACK SUGGESTIONS

Children are often very hungry after school so a light snack of a variation of the lunch suggestions would be appropriate.

WHEN EATING OUT

In restaurants, choose a grill or roast dish with hot vegetables, or specify a salad without dressing, followed by fresh fruit or fresh fruit salad.

When caught out, and everyone is buying take-away food, the safest foods are barbecued chicken (without eating the skin), fried fish (without eating the batter) or a steak sandwich (without eating the bread).

BREAD SUBSTITUTES

As bread is probably the single most difficult sacrifice to make when undertaking an anti-Candida diet, the alternatives are listed first. All contain carbohydrate, so may be consumed only in moderation.

rice cakes (commercially available), 2 rice cakes equals 1 M serve.

rice crispbread, 2 crispbread equals 1 M serve.

some cruskits (check packet for yeast content) 2 equals 1 M serve.

some crispbreads (check for yeast content) 2 equals 1 M serve.

pancakes.

damper.

soda bread.

potato cake.

BASIC PANCAKES   M

1 cup wholemeal plain flour
1 egg
1 cup milk
pinch salt

Sift the flour and salt and gradually work in egg and half the milk, beat well for one minute and add remainder of milk. Allow to stand for 30 minutes to produce a lighter batter. Add sufficient quantity to a hot pan greased with butter, margarine or oil and cook both sides to a light brown colour. Serve with fruit or savoury filling or make variations as for BUCKWHEAT PANCAKES.

BUCKWHEAT PANCAKES M

1 cup buckwheat flour
1 cup maize meal
1 egg
1½ cups milk or water

Mix together the dry ingredients and stir in the egg and half the liquid until smooth. Beat well while adding the remainder of the liquid. Pour sufficient into a hot pan, greased with butter, margarine or oil and cook well on both sides. Serve hot with freshly stewed apple, apricots or peaches, or a savoury filling. Pancakes may be frozen and served freshly thawed as a bread substitute or with a savoury filling.

Variations:
Substitute rice or potato flour for maize meal.
Add a mashed banana, a grated apple or 2 tablespoons of ground hazelnuts to the batter mixture.

CORN BREAD M

1 cup maize meal
½ cup soy flour
¼ cup oatmeal
1 cup milk
¼ cup skim milk powder
1 egg
½ level teaspoon salt
2 level teaspoons baking powder

Mix the dry ingredients. Mix powdered milk into the milk and mix into the dry ingredients along with the egg. Place in a greased loaf tin and bake in an oven pre-heated to 190°C (375°F) for about 30 minutes.

COCONUT PANCAKES   M

1 cup coconut
1 cup soy or rice flour, or maize meal
3 teaspoons baking powder
½ teaspoon salt
2 tablespoons oil
2 cups water

Place all ingredients into blender and blend until just mixed.
Pour sufficient into a hot pan greased with butter, margarine
or oil and cook both sides.

POTATO PANCAKES   M

2 medium potatoes, cooked, mashed and still warm
1 tablespoons maize meal
pinch of salt
1 tablespoonful of butter, margarine or oil

Stir butter or oil into potato and then add dry ingredients to
provide a soft, dry consistency. Roll onto a floured surface
to desired thickness. Cut into circles, prick all over and place
in a hot pan greased with butter or oil and cook both sides.
Serve hot as a basis for scrambled eggs or other savoury fillings
or cold as a bread substitute.

POTATO CAKES   M

2 medium potatoes, grated
1 small onion, chopped (optional)

Mix potato and onion and place sufficient quantity into a hot pan of approx. 1 tablespoonful of butter, margarine or oil and cook on both sides.

COTTAGE CHEESE PANCAKES   M

1 cup cottage cheese
1 egg
1 tablespoon oil
½ cup wholemeal plain flour
¼ cup white flour
1 tablespoon skim milk powder
½ cup water

Beat the egg and blend in the cottage cheese and add remaining ingredients. Pour sufficient batter into a hot pan greased with butter, margarine or oil and cook both sides until brown. Serve hot or cold as for BUCKWHEAT PANCAKES.

DAMPER   M

3 cups wholemeal self raising flour
2 teaspoons baking powder
1 to 1½ cups warm milk

Mix the dry ingredients and add warm milk to form a scone-type dough. Kneed lightly and place in a greased loaf tin. Place in an oven pre-heated to 230°C (450°F), reset to 200° (400°F) and bake until done, approximately 30 minutes.

SODA BREAD

2 cups wholemeal plain flour
⅓ cup water
⅓ cup milk
½ level teaspoon salt
½ level teaspoon Bicarbonate of Soda
1 level teaspoon Cream of Tartar

Sift dry ingredients and make into a dough with the liquids.
Quickly form into round flat loaf and place on a greased baking
tray. Cover loaf with a deep 6 or 7 inch cake tin, and bake
in 230°C (450°F) oven for 30 minutes. Remove tin and leave
loaf in oven for a further 10-15 minutes to brown.

RICE BREAD   M

2 cups rice flour
¾ cup water
2 tablespoons butter, margarine or oil
½ level teaspoon salt
½ level teaspoon Cream of Tartar

Mix and sift dry ingredients. Melt butter or margarine, mix
with water and stir into dry ingredients. Place in a greased
loaf tin and bake in an oven pre-heated to 190°C (375°F) for
about 30 minutes.

APPETISERS

Dips can be used as an appetiser with sticks of fresh carrot or celery or with blanched beans, snow peas, broccoli, cauliflower or asparagus. They can also be used as a spread for pancakes or bread substitutes.

SALMON DIP   N

1½ cups ricotta cheese
1 can salmon (170gr., drained)
1 tablespoon chopped spring onions
1 teaspoon lemon juice
pinch cayenne pepper
pinch salt

Thoroughly mix all the ingredients together and serve in a small bowl. Garnish with parsley or chopped spring onions.

AVOCADO DIP   N

2 avocados
1 large tomato
4 teaspoons lemon juice
1 tablespoon chopped spring onions
1 clove garlic (crushed)

Thoroughly mix together the peeled and mashed avocado, the peeled and chopped tomato and the other ingredients and serve in a small bowl. Garnish with parsley or chopped spring onions.

RICOTTA DIP   L

1½ cups ricotta cheese
½ cup skim milk
1 teaspoon vanilla essence
1 tablespoon grated lemon rind

Beat the cheese, vanilla and lemon rind together until smooth.
Slowly add the skim milk while beating. Serve in a bowl
surrounded with slices of fresh apple, peaches, apricots,
strawberries or pineapple. Garnish with a sprig of mint.

CUCUMBER DIP   L

1 small cucumber
1 cup low-fat natural yoghurt
2 cloves garlic (crushed)
1 teaspoon lemon juice
1 teaspoon mint (chopped)

Peel and grate cucumbers and allow to drain. Combine other
ingredients and fold in the cucumber. Serve chilled in a small
bowl. Garnish with a sprig of mint.

SALMON AND CUCUMBER SPREAD   N

1 can salmon (170gr. drained)
1 small cucumber (peeled and seeded)
½ small capsicum (seeded)
1 teaspoon lemon juice

Mix together all the ingredients in a blender or food processor. Pour into small bowl and refrigerate. Serve chilled. Garnish with parsley.

TAHINI SPROUT SPREAD   L

1 cup non-fat natural yoghurt
½ cup tahini
1 teaspoon lemon juice
¾ cup alfalfa sprouts
1 clove garlic (crushed)

Mix together all the ingredients and refrigerate. Serve chilled.

STUFFED EGGS   L

6 eggs, hard boiled
1 tablespoon chives, snipped
1 tablespoon parsley, chopped
2 tablespoons low fat natural yoghurt
¼ teaspoon curry powder
2 teaspoons lemon juice
cayenne pepper to taste
salt and pepper to taste

Peel eggs and cut in half lengthwise. Remove yolks and mix with the remaining ingredients. Carefully spoon back into the hollowed whites, chill and serve garnished with cayenne pepper or parsley.

SOUPS

The following selection of recipes will provide a basis for a variety of soups for all seasons. Most have low or negligible carbohydrate content, so can be eaten quite freely and also may be frozen and quickly re-heated for a quick meal.

CUCUMBER SOUP   N

3 cups freshly prepared chicken stock (see recipe)
1 medium cucumber
2 spring onions
1 tablespoon butter or margarine
½ cup white flour
¼ teaspoon salt
¼ cup yoghurt
1 egg yolk
pepper to taste

Seed and cut cucumber into 1 inch cubes, combine with the chopped onions and the chicken stock in a large saucepan. Cover and simmer for 30 minutes or until the cucumber is soft. Push through a sieve and discard skins. Melt the butter or margarine in a large saucepan, stir in the flour and cook for 1 minute. Remove the pan from the heat and gradually add the cucumber stock. Stir continuously until the soup boils and thickens, add salt and pepper to taste. Combine the yoghurt and egg yolk and stir through the soup.

Serve chilled or hot, garnished with thin slices of cucumber.

CHICKEN STOCK   N

1 large chicken or 500gr. chicken wings
3 cups hot water
1 medium carrot
1 medium onion
3 sticks celery
pepper to taste

Coarsely chop vegetables and combine with other ingredients in a large saucepan. Cover and simmer for 2-3 hours. Allow to cool and place in refrigerator to chill to facilitate removal of fat. Strain and use immediately or store in freezer.

BEEF STOCK   N

500gr. shin beef
1 medium carrot
1 medium onion
3 sticks celery
pepper or peppercorns to taste

Coarsely chop vegetables and combine with other ingredients in a large saucepan. Cover and simmer for 3 hours. Allow to cool, remove fat, strain and use immediately or store in freezer.

MINESTRONE   M

½ cup borlotti beans, soaked overnight
2 cups beef stock
1 medium carrot, diced
2 sticks celery, sliced
1 leek, sliced
1 medium onion, sliced
1 clove garlic, crushed
½ cup cabbage, shredded
2 large, ripe tomatoes
2 tablespoons oil
salt and pepper to taste

Drain beans and place in pan with 1 cup beef stock, bring slowly to boil and simmer for 30 minutes. Heat oil in a pan and add carrots, celery and onion, cover and cook for five minutes. Add second cup of stock and bring to boil, add leeks and tomatoes and simmer gently for 30 minutes. Add cabbage and garlic and cook gently until the vegetables are thoroughly cooked, season to taste. Serve hot.

PUMPKIN SOUP   L

500 gr. pumpkin, peeled and diced
1 medium onion, finely chopped
1 cup chicken stock
1 cup milk
1 teaspoon oil
¼ teaspoon freshly grated nutmeg
salt and pepper to taste

Heat oil in pan, add onion, cover and cook for 10 minutes. Add chicken stock and bring to boil. Add pumpkin and simmer for 30 minutes. Allow to cool sufficiently to puree in blender or food processor to a smooth consistency. Return to pan, add remaining ingredients and heat gently until ready to serve. Serve with a dob of yoghurt or garnish with a sprig of parsley or chopped chives.

ZUCCHINI SOUP   N

3 medium zucchini, thickly sliced
1 small onion, chopped
1 small potato, scrubbed and thinly sliced
1 teaspoon oil
2 cups chicken stock
½ teaspoon dried tarragon
salt and pepper to taste

Heat oil in pan, add vegetables and tarragon, salt and ground pepper. Cover and cook for 10 minutes. Add stock, cover and simmer for 20 minutes. Allow to cool sufficiently to puree in blender or food processor. Serve hot or cold with a dob of yoghurt or a squeeze of lemon juice.

TOMATO SOUP   N

1 kg. ripe tomatoes
2 medium onions
2 large carrots
1 stick celery
2 cups beef stock
3 cloves garlic (crushed)
1 tablespoon oil
1 bay leaf
¼ teaspoon marjoram
¼ teaspoon mixed herbs
½ teaspoon salt
pepper to taste

Coarsely chop all vegetables. Heat the oil in a large saucepan and add the onion and garlic and cook until the onion is soft. Add all the remaining ingredients and simmer gently for 45 minutes. Cool and puree in blender or food processor. Serve hot, garnished with sprig of parsley or mint or stir in a teaspoon of yoghurt.

CHILLED TOMATO SOUP   N

500 gr. ripe tomatoes, peeled and chopped
1 medium cucumber, chopped
1 green or red pepper, chopped
2 cups water
2 cloves garlic (crushed)
2 tablespoons oil
salt and pepper to taste

Mix all the ingredients together in a blender or food processor and puree. Serve chilled garnished with finely chopped chives.

SALADS AND SALAD DRESSINGS

MAYONNAISE   N

1 cup oil
2 egg yolks
2 teaspoons lemon juice
½ teaspoon salt
½ teaspoon mustard powder
freshly ground pepper to taste

Place egg yolks, salt, lemon juice, mustard and pepper in a
mixing bowl and whisk until smooth. Ensure the oil is at room
temperature and slowly add to the egg mixture drop by drop
with continuous whisking. As the mixture thickens, the oil may
be added more quickly while whisking.

COTTAGE CHEESE DRESSING   N

1 cup cottage cheese
¾ cup soured cream (see recipe)
1 clove garlic, crushed
2 teaspoons lemon juice
1 teaspoon mustard powder
½ teaspoon salt
freshly ground pepper to taste

Place all the ingredients in a blender or food processor and
blend until smooth. Serve chilled. This dressing may be used
as a substitute for mayonnaise.

FRENCH DRESSING   N

2 tablespoons oil
2 tablespoons lemon juice
½ teaspoon mustard powder
1 clove garlic, crushed
¼ teaspoon freshly ground pepper

Place all ingredients in a screw top jar and shake well. Serve chilled.

ORANGE COLESLAW   L

2 oranges, peeled and segmented
½ cabbage, finely shredded
1 green pepper, finely sliced
1 red pepper, finely sliced
2 teaspoons lemon juice
½ teaspoon grated lemon rind
1 cup mayonnaise

Combine all the ingredients in a large bowl and chill well before serving.

CUCUMBER SALAD   N

2 medium cucumbers
1 cup chopped celery
1 cup chopped cold, cooked lean meat, chicken or fish
½ cup chopped radish
½ cup French dressing

Cut cucumbers lengthwise, take out some of the pulp and combine with other ingredients to use as stuffing for cucumber cases. Garnish with a sprig of parsley.

COLESLAW   L

2 carrots, grated
½ cabbage, finely shredded
½ cup spring onions, finely chopped
1 red apple, finely chopped
1 cup fresh pineapple, finely diced
1 teaspoon lemon juice
½ cup toasted almonds
½ cup yoghurt dressing

Combine all the ingredients in a large bowl and chill well before serving.

AVOCADO AND MELON SALAD   N

2 medium avocados, halved and stoned
½ medium honeydew melon, seeded.
1 tablespoon lemon juice
¾ cup French dressing

Scoop out the avocado flesh with a melon baller, place in bowl and sprinkle with lemon juice. Scoop out the melon flesh in the same way and add to the avocado balls. Chill 2 or 3 hours. Just before serving, pour over the dressing and gently toss the ingredients until well coated.

YOGHURT DRESSING L

½ cup natural yoghurt
½ cup oil
2 tablespoons lemon juice
¼ cup chopped chives
¼ cup chopped parsley
1 clove garlic, crushed
½ teaspoon mustard powder
½ teaspoon salt
freshly ground pepper to taste

Place all ingredients in a blender or food processor and blend until smooth. Transfer to a jar and refrigerate until serving.

CUCUMBER DRESSING L

1 cup natural yoghurt
4 teaspoons lemon juice
1 cup cucumber, coarsely grated
1 teaspoon chopped parsley
freshly ground pepper to taste

Combine all the ingredients in a jar and shake. Serve chilled as a salad dressing or as a dip for blanched vegetables, or on jacket baked potato.

CURRIED RICE SALAD   M

1 cup cooked brown rice
1 medium red apple, chopped
¼ cup walnuts, chopped
½ cup red or green pepper, finely sliced
3 teaspoons curry powder
2 tablespoons oil
2 teaspoons lemon juice

Mix together the oil, lemon juice and curry as the dressing. Pour over the rice while still warm and mix well. Allow to cool and add the other ingredients and toss lightly. Serve well chilled.

TOMATO SALAD WITH GINGER   N

4 medium tomatoes, coarsely chopped
1 small onion, finely chopped
1 teaspoon fresh ginger, finely chopped
2 tablespoons lemon juice
2 tablespoons parsley, finely chopped
1 tablespoon chives, snipped

Combine all ingredients except parsley, mix gently and chill before serving. Garnish with the chopped parsley.

CHICKEN SALAD WITH RICE   L

1 cup cold cooked brown rice
2 cups cold lean chicken, chopped
½ cucumber, sliced
1 medium onion, finely chopped
½ green pepper, finely sliced
1 cob corn, cook and remove kernels with a sharp knife
4 tablespoons French dressing
½ cup yoghurt dressing
1 tablespoon chives, snipped

Combine all ingredients, except chives, mix gently and chill before serving. Garnish with snipped chives.

TOSSED SALAD   N

1 medium lettuce
1 clove garlic
6 spring onions, finely sliced
½ green pepper, finely sliced
½ red pepper, finely sliced
4 medium tomatoes, chopped coarsely
1 cucumber, sliced
½ cup French dressing

Rub a wooden bowl with the clove of garlic, break up the lettuce and combine with onions and toss. Arrange peppers, tomato and cucumber on top and add the French dressing.

PRAWN AND AVOCADO SALAD   L

1 kg cooked fresh prawns
2 avocados, balled or diced
2 medium carrots, cut into strips
1 small lettuce or Chinese cabbage, finely shredded
1 spring onion, chopped
2 sticks celery, cut into strips
1 tablespoon roasted sesame seeds
1 cup French dressing

Combine all the ingredients in a large bowl, toss lightly and chill well before serving.

ORIENTAL SALAD   M

1 cup bean or alfalfa sprouts
1 cup cooked brown rice
2 sticks celery, finely sliced
2 cups cooked lean chicken or pork
½ cup toasted almonds
3 spring onions, chopped
1 medium carrot, grated
½ green pepper, chopped
¾ cup French dressing

Combine all ingredients in a large bowl, toss lightly and chill well before serving. Garnish with chopped parsley.

POTATO SALAD   M

4 medium potatoes, cooked and diced
1 small onion, finely chopped
1 stick celery, sliced
1 cup cooked fresh peas
½ teaspoon mustard powder
freshly ground pepper to taste
2 tablespoons parsley, finely chopped
1 cup yoghurt dressing

Combine all the ingredients in a large bowl, toss lightly and chill well before serving.

MACARONI SALAD   M

2 cups macaroni, cooked
½ medium cucumber, sliced
2 medium tomatoes, coarsely chopped
2 sticks celery, sliced
2 cups cooked cold lean meat or chicken
½ cup French dressing

Combine the ingredients in a large bowl, toss lightly and chill well before serving on a bed of lettuce. Garnish with chopped parsley.

MAIN COURSES

OSSO BUCO N

4 veal knuckles or shanks (cut into 2 inch pieces)
2 tablespoons butter or margarine
2 carrots, chopped
2 large onions, finely chopped
3 sticks celery
2 cloves garlic, crushed
flour
salt and pepper to taste
2 tablespoons oil
2 400 gr. cans whole tomatoes
2 cups beef stock
1 teaspoon thyme
1 bay leaf
1 teaspoon basil
1 teaspoon grated lemon rind
3 tablespoons parsley, chopped

Heat half the butter and add carrots, onions and celery and one clove of garlic. Remove from heat and transfer to a large casserole dish. Coat the pieces of shank with flour seasoned with salt and pepper and cook in remaining heated butter and oil until brown on all sides. Pack the shanks on top of the vegetables (upright to retain the marrow). Push the tomatoes and their liquid through a sieve. Bring to boil with beef stock, basil, thyme and bay leaf, and season with salt and pepper. Pour sauce over veal shanks, cover and bake in a moderate oven until veal is tender. Sprinkle over the remaining garlic, parsley and lemon rind.

LOW CARBOHYDRATE TOMATO SAUCE   N

4 large ripe tomatoes
1 medium onion, chopped
salt and pepper to taste.

Cook the tomatoes and onions over moderate heat until soft, season and cook further to reduce to desired consistency. May be used fresh or may be frozen for future use.

HAMBURGERS   N

500 gr. lean ground beef
1 medium carrot, grated
4 spring onions, chopped
1 green pepper, chopped
1 egg, beaten
1 tablespoon low carbohydrate tomato sauce (see recipe below)
salt and pepper to taste

Combine the ingredients, form into patties and cook on a barbecue or grill.

SOUVLAKI   N

1 kg. lamb, cubed
1 tablespoon rosemary, chopped
1 teaspoon salt

Thread the lamb cubes onto skewers and roll in the rosemary and salt. Cook on a barbecue or grill.

CHICKEN YOGHURT L

4 large chicken breasts, boned
1 cup natural yoghurt
1 clove garlic, crushed
2 spring onions, sliced lengthwise
1 tablespoon parsley, chopped
¼ teaspoon chilli powder
¼ teaspoon cinnamon
¼ teaspoon ginger
1 teaspoon salt

Arrange the chicken breasts and onions in a baking dish.
Combine the remaining ingredients and pour over the chicken
and allow to marinate for several hours. Place in an oven,
preheated to 180°C (350°F) and bake for 90 minutes.

ROAST CHICKEN WITH ORANGE N

1 medium chicken
2 oranges
1 clove garlic
3 tablespoons oil

Juice one orange and put the juice aside. Prepare the chicken
and rub the outside skin with the orange rind. Stuff the chicken
with the other orange, quartered, and the garlic clove. Brush
the outside with the oil and bake for one hour at 180°C (350°F).
Pour over the orange juice and bake for a further 45 minutes.

CHICKEN CROQUETTES   M

2 cups cooked chicken (chopped)
2 tablespoons plain wholemeal flour
1 cup skim milk
1½ tablespoons butter, margarine or oil
1 tablespoon parsley, chopped

Melt the butter and stir in the flour and cook over a low heat
for 1 minute. Remove from heat and mix in the skim milk and
cook until thick. Spread the chopped chicken on a large plate
and pour over the hot sauce. Allow to cool and then chill well.
Form into croquettes and bake in an oven, preheated to 180°C
(350°F) until crisp and brown.

CHICKEN RISOTTO   M

1 cup brown rice, cooked
1 tablespoon oil
1 clove garlic, crushed
1 cup cooked chicken, chopped
2 tomatoes, chopped
½ each of green, red and yellow pepper, chopped
½ teaspoon salt
freshly ground pepper to taste

Heat the oil in a pan and lightly cook the garlic, chicken,
peppers and tomatoes. Add a little water and the salt and
pepper and cook until vegetables are soft, stirring frequently.
Add the hot, cooked rice and serve. Garnish with parsley.

SALMON AND ONION PANCAKE FILLING   L

1 medium tin salmon
1 cup milk
3 tablespoons butter or margarine
3 tablespoons wholemeal flour
1 medium onion, chopped
½ stick celery, chopped
2 teaspoons lemon juice
salt and pepper to taste

Melt the butter in a saucepan, stir in the flour and add salt and pepper. Slowly add 1 cup milk, stirring to form a smooth sauce. Drain and flake the salmon and fold into the sauce. Add the onions, celery and lemon juice. Serve with suitable pancakes.

WHITING AND POTATOES   M

4 small fillets of whiting or other fish
1 medium onion, sliced
3 medium potatoes, thinly sliced
1 tablespoon wholemeal flour
3 medium tomatoes, coarsely chopped
2 tablespoons oil
1 teaspoon salt
freshly ground black pepper

Heat the oil in a large pan and saute the onions and potato for 10 minutes. Stir in the flour and add the tomatoes, salt and pepper to taste. Cover and cook for 20 minutes. Place the fish fillets on top of the potatoes, recover and cook until the fish is cooked.

WHITING KEBABS

N

1 kg. whiting fillets
2 medium onions, finely chopped
1 cup lemon juice
3 bay leaves
¼ teaspoon cumin
3 large tomatoes, quartered
2 large green peppers

Cube the fish, place in dish and sprinkle with onions and lemon juice. Add bay leaves and cumin and allow to marinate in refrigerator for 1 hour. Thread the fish cubes, tomato pieces and squares of green pepper onto skewers, brush lightly with oil and cook under grill or on barbecue until fish is cooked. Serve with slices of lemon.

WHITING WITH GINGER

N

4 whiting fillets
3 tablespoons butter or margarine
3 medium onions, thickly sliced
3 medium tomatoes, sliced
1 tablespoon lemon juice
1 tablespoon grated fresh green ginger
salt and pepper to taste

Place fish fillets in a greased baking dish. Melt the butter or margarine and add the ginger, lemon juice, salt and pepper and pour over the fish. Cover with alternate layers of slices of onion and tomato. Place in an oven preheated to 180°C (350°F) and bake for 25 minutes. Baste frequently. Garnish with chopped parsley or chives.

BAKED SNAPPER   N

1 whole snapper of approx. 1.5kg.
1 medium onion, finely chopped
1 stick celery, chopped
½ cup spring onions, chopped
½ green pepper, chopped
1 tablespoon grated green ginger
1½ cups cooked brown rice
1 tablespoon butter or margarine
¼ cup lemon juice
salt and pepper to taste
1 lemon, thinly sliced

Mix together onion, celery, green pepper, salt and pepper and stuff into the fish. Place the fish in a well greased baking dish. Melt the butter in a saucepan, remove from heat and add lemon juice, ginger, spring onions and salt and pepper. Pour sauce over fish and bake in an oven pre-heated to 180°C (350°F) for 45 minutes. Baste frequently. Place fish in a hot serving dish, pour over juices and garnish with slices of lemon and sprigs of parsley.

TROUT WITH ALMONDS   N

4 medium sized trout
3 tablespoons flour
1 teaspoon salt
3 tablespoons butter or margarine
½ cup almond flakes
¼ cup lemon juice
1 tablespoon chopped parsley
freshly ground black pepper to taste

Coat the fish with the seasoned flour. Heat half the butter in a pan and cook the trout until brown, keep warm. Heat the remaining butter until boiling, add the almonds and cook until golden brown. Add the lemon juice and boil away most of the lemon juice while stirring continuously. Stir in the parsley and pour over the trout in a serving dish. Garnish with a light sprinkling of flaked almonds.

WHITING WITH VEGETABLE RICE   M

2 cups cooked brown rice
4 small whiting fillets
1½ cups cooked vegetables (peas, carrots, beans, celery)
2 tablespoons butter or margarine
salt and pepper to taste

Poach the fish in water for 10 minutes. Flake the fish and combine with the other ingredients. Melt the butter in a large pan and lightly cook the rice mixture until starting to brown.

SALMON LOAF   L

1 medium can salmon in brine/water
1 medium onion, finely chopped
¼ cup lemon juice
1 green pepper, chopped
1 stick celery, chopped
skim milk
pinch cayenne pepper
1 egg white
2 tablespoons oatmeal

Drain liquid from salmon and make up to ½ cup with skim milk. Mix all the ingredients together, place in an oiled loaf tin and bake in an oven at 180°C (350°F) for 1 hour.

LEMON WHITING   N

4 fillets of whiting or other fish
1 tablespoon butter or margarine
½ teaspoon grated lemon rind
juice of 1 lemon
freshly ground black pepper

Sprinkle fillets with pepper and place on grill tray. Mix together the butter, lemon juice and rind and spread half over the fish. Grill until lightly browned, turn over and spread balance of butter mixture and grill until cooked. Garnish with slices of lemon or sprigs of parsley.

TUNA STUFFED PEPPERS   M

4 green peppers, halved and seeded
1 small can tuna, drained
2½ cups cooked brown rice
1 medium onion, chopped
1 teaspoon butter or margarine
½ teaspoon thyme
1 cup cottage cheese
½ cup tomato sauce
1 tablespoon lemon juice

Blanch the pepper halves in boiling water for 5 minutes, drain. Saute the onion in the butter until golden brown and add to the rice with the cottage cheese, tomato sauce, thyme, lemon juice and tuna. Bake in an oven at 180°C (350°) for 30 minutes.

SAUCES

Most sauces have a medium to high carbohydrate content so are not ideal as constituents of the anti-Candida diet. However, if used only as a dressing for a dish in small quantities they will not contribute a large amount of carbohydrate to the overall diet.

WHITE SAUCE

1 cup skim milk
2 tablespoons cornflour
salt and pepper to taste

Make a thin paste of the cornflour and a small amount of the milk. Bring the balance of the milk almost to the boil. Add the paste and beat well. Add the salt and pepper.

ALTERNATIVE WHITE SAUCE

1½ tablespoons butter
1 cup skim milk
1 tablespoon flour
salt and pepper to taste

Melt the butter in a small saucepan, stir in the flour and cook for 2 minutes. Remove from heat and slowly add milk while stirring continuously. Bring to boil while stirring and boil until the sauce thickens to the desired consistency.

Either of these sauces can be used as a basis for various sauces by the addition of chopped chives or parsley or mint or some sauteed onions.

YOGHURT SAUCE

1 cup natural yoghurt
½ tablespoon cumin
1 tablespoon lemon juice
freshly ground pepper to taste

Mix together all the ingredients and refrigerate until required. Yoghurt sauce is suitable for use as a dressing for a cold salad such as potato salad.

HOME MADE SOUR CREAM

1 cup cottage cheese
½ cup low-fat natural yoghurt

Combine the ingredients in a blender or food processor until smooth. This may be used as a substitute for sour cream on hot potatoes with a sprinkling of chopped cooked bacon.

VEGETABLE DISHES

TOMATO RICOTTA   N

4 large tomatoes, halved
2 tablespoons chives, chopped
½ teaspoon salt
1 cup ricotta cheese
freshly ground black pepper

Blend the chives, ricotta cheese and salt and pepper and pile onto tomato halves to give stuffed tomato appearance. Serve on a bed of lettuce.

POTATO AND CABBAGE CASSEROLE   M

4 large potatoes, boiled and sliced
2 large apples, peeled and sliced
2 large onions, sliced
500 gr. cabbage, shredded
1 cup cottage cheese
salt and pepper to taste
cabbage leaves, blanched for 2 minutes or until pliable

Line a casserole dish with blanched cabbage leaves and add the layers of onion, cabbage, apple and potato. Cover with cottage cheese and sprinkle with salt and pepper. Repeat layers until complete and finish with a layer of potato. Cover and cook for 40 minutes. Remove cover and continue cooking until potatoes are browned.

ZUCCHINI IN TOMATO SAUCE   N

8 small zucchini, thickly sliced
3 medium tomatoes, chopped
1 clove garlic, crushed
½ teaspoon basil
freshly ground black pepper

Place the tomatoes in a saucepan with the garlic, basil and pepper and cook until soft. Mash the tomato mixture, add the zucchini and cook until soft. Serve hot as an accompaniment to a meat dish.

SPINACH AND RICOTTA FLAN   N

1 bunch spinach, chopped
1½ cups ricotta cheese
2 eggs
¼ cup skim milk powder
½ cup freshly prepared tomato juice
2 tablespoons parsley, chopped
2 medium onions, sliced
freshly ground black pepper

Gently boil the spinach for 5 minutes, drain and cool. Beat together the eggs, milk powder, ricotta cheese, tomato juice, parsley and pepper in a blender or food processor until smooth. Oil a small casserole dish and line with spinach leaves and pour in the egg and ricotta mixture. Cook onion in a little water until soft and arrange on the egg and ricotta mixture. Bake in an oven heated to 150°C (300°F) for 45 minutes.

HOT POTATO SALAD   M

3 medium potatoes, chopped coarsely
1 medium onion, finely chopped
1 red pepper, finely chopped
1 green pepper, finely chopped
1 stick celery, finely chopped
1 medium carrot, grated
½ cup mayonnaise
freshly ground black pepper

Cook potatoes until tender and mix in the other vegetables. Place in an oiled casserole dish, pour over the mayonnaise and cook in an oven at 180°C (350°F) for 20 minutes.

RATATOUILLE   N

1 green pepper, seeded and cut into rings
1 small eggplant, sliced
2 zucchini, sliced
½ tablespoon oil
1 clove garlic, crushed
2 medium onions, sliced
2 medium tomatoes, sliced

Heat the oil in a large pan and add the garlic, pepper, eggplant, onion and zucchini. Cover and simmer for 10 minutes, add tomato and simmer for a further 10 minutes uncovered.

POTATOES AND ONIONS L

3 large potatoes, thinly sliced
1 large onion, sliced into rings
¾ cup skim milk
freshly ground black pepper

Oil a shallow casserole dish and layer potatoes and onions. Pour over the skim milk, sprinkle with pepper and cook in an oven at 180°C (350°F) for 1½ hours.

BEANS AND TOMATOES M

2 medium onions, chopped
4 medium tomatoes, chopped
2 cloves garlic, crushed
1 tablespoon oil
½ teaspoon fresh basil
1 bay leaf
1½ cups cooked kidney beans

Add the oil to a pan and cook onion rings, add tomatoes and garlic and cook until mixture is smooth. Add the basil, bay leaf and pepper. Drain and add the beans, cover and simmer for 20 minutes. Garnish with a sprig of parsley.

DESSERTS

Most dessert recipes are *high* in carbohydrate because most contain sugar. For that reason, the ideal dessert is a serve of fresh fruit. However, for that special occasion or for extra interest, the following recipes may suit.

FRUITY PANCAKES

2 large cooking apples, sliced
1 cup skim milk
3 eggs
½ cup wholemeal flour
2 teaspoons vanilla essence

Place the apple slices in an oiled pie dish or casserole dish. Combine the remaining ingredients in a blender or processor until smooth, pour over apple and bake in an oven preheated to 350 degrees for 40 minutes. Serve with HOME MADE SOUR CREAM.

As an alternative, substitute fresh apricots, peaches, pears or strawberries.

COTTAGE CHEESE PANCAKES

1 cup cottage cheese
¾ cup wholemeal flour
1 egg
1 tablespoon oil
1 tablespoon skim milk powder
½ cup water

Combine egg, cottage cheese and oil in blender or food processor and slowly add other ingredients. Pour sufficient batter into a hot, oiled pan and cook until golden brown. Turn and cook other side. Serve with freshly stewed fruit or STRAWBERRY JAM or STRAWBERRY TOPPING.

STRAWBERRY JAM

250gr. fresh strawberries
4 granny smith apples, peeled and cored
2 cups freshly squeezed orange juice
1 teaspoon cinnamon
rind of 1 orange

Grate the apple and add to the washed strawberries in a saucepan. Add the remaining ingredients and slowly bring to the boil and simmer for 40 minutes or until thick, stirring occasionally. Pour into sterilized jars, cool and seal.
Refrigerate after opening

STRAWBERRY TOPPING

1 cup ricotta cheese
½ cup non fat natural yoghurt
1 cup strawberries, chopped

Mix cheese and yoghurt until smooth. Stir in the strawberries and serve with pancakes.

FRUIT SORBET

2 cups fresh strawberries, apricot, peach or other fruit, chopped
2 cups carrot, finely sliced

Cook carrot until soft. Stew fruit until soft. Combine in a blender until smooth, add lemon juice and freeze in casserole dish, stirring frequently to break up the ice crystals.

YOGHURT FRUIT DESSERT

2 cups non fat natural yoghurt
4 passionfruit pulp
1 cup fresh pineapple pieces
2 bananas, sliced

Combine all the ingredients in a bowl and stir together well. Serve chilled in individual fruit bowls.

FRUIT JELLY

1 cup boiling water
3 teaspoons gelatine
1 cup freshly squeezed orange juice
1 teaspoon grated orange rind
1 cup stewed fresh pineapple

Dissolve the gelatine in the boiling water. Stir in juice and rind and allow to almost set. Fold in the pineapple and refrigerate.

WAFFLES

1 cup soy beans
1¼ cups oatmeal
1½ cups water
1 tablespoon oil

Place the soy beans in a dish, add sufficient water to cover and leave to soak overnight. Drain and combine with other ingredients in a blender until light and airy. Pour into preheated waffle iron and cook for 15 minutes at medium setting. Do not open waffle iron for 15 minutes. Serve with fresh or stewed fruit.

BANANA PANCAKES

1 cup wholemeal flour
1 banana, mashed
½ teaspoon lemon juice
1 teaspoon grated lemon rind
skim milk

Combine all ingredients, stirring in the milk to obtain a smooth paste. Drop spoonfuls onto a hot pan or skillet. Turn to cook the other side when bubbles appear on the top.

BEVERAGES

FRUIT PUNCH

2 cups low calorie dry ginger ale
4 cups low calorie lemonade
juice of 2 lemons
pulp of 4 passionfruit
1 tablespoon chopped mint
1 lemon, thinly sliced
6 drops Angostura Bitters

Combine the ingredients in a large bowl or jug just before serving.

SUMMER FIZZ

½ cup freshly squeezed lemon or orange juice
1 cup mineral water

Combine ingredients and pour over ice in serving glasses

FRUITY DELIGHT

1 cup buttermilk
1 cup freshly squeezed orange juice

Combine ingredients in a blender until smooth. Serve chilled.

STRAWBERRY DELIGHT

1 cup buttermilk
1 cup strawberries

Combine ingredients in a blender until smooth. Serve chilled.

WATERMELON SURPRISE

3 cups watermelon balls or cubes
2 cups ice cubes
1 sprig mint

Combine all ingredients in a blender until light and frothy.

SNACKS AND CAKES

WHOLEMEAL SCONES

1 cup wholemeal self raising flour
1 cup self raising flour
1½ cups tablespoons butter or margarine
½ cup skim milk
½ cup water

Combine the flours and fold in the butter with fingertips to form a fine crumbly mixture. Mix in sufficient milk and water to make a soft dough. Roll out on a floured board and cut into scones. Place on an oiled baking tray and cook in a hot oven for 15 minutes.

WHOLEMEAL PASTRY

1 cup wholemeal plain flour
½ cup self raising flour
1 teaspoon baking powder
2 tablespoons butter or margarine
1 cup iced water
2 teaspons lemon juice

Combine dry ingredients and rub in the butter as for scones. Add sufficient water and lemon juice to form a stiff dough. Knead into a ball, refrigerate and use as desired.

BANANA LOAF

1 egg
4 tablespoons butter or margarine
1 cup grated carrot
2 ripe bananas, mashed
1½ cups wholemeal plain flour
1 teaspoon bicarb. soda
½ teaspoon cinnamon

Beat together the egg and margarine, fold in the carrot and bananas. Stir in the dry ingredients and mix well. Pour into an oiled loaf tin and bake in an oven at 150°C (300°F) for one and a half hours.

CHAPTER 10

VITAMIN
AND MINERAL
SUPPLEMENTS

An adequate supply of vitamins and minerals should be provided by the consumption of a well balanced, varied diet of freshly gathered foods. However, if the foods are not fresh, or your diet is restricted, or your nutrient absorption is disturbed by Candida, or your chemical load is heavier than normal, then you may find that you may be helped by supplementing your diet with commercially available supplements of vitamins and minerals. Some people find that extra vitamins help them through their allergic reactions.

Vitamins and minerals are substances which cannot be manufactured within the body and so must be obtained from food sources. They are the building blocks of some of the more important hormones and enzymes which keep the body functioning. It is important, when choosing a nutritional supplement, to ensure that the preparation is free of any potentially allergenic material such as: yeast, sugar, chemicals, artificial colouring or flavouring, or derivatives of foods to which you are allergic such as: wheat, dairy, soy or corn.

The whole range of vitamins, minerals and essential fatty acids are necessary for normal functioning of the body. In chronic Candidiasis and other allergy conditions, some vitamins are more important because either absorption is altered, or more is needed by the body to deal with Candida toxins. The more important supplements are:

PYRIDOXINE (VITAMIN B6)

Pyridoxine has been established as an important basic raw material for the establishment of a competent immune system (and some more recent research by Dr Orion Truss has suggested that Candida toxins are great consumers of pyridoxine.)

PANTOTHENIC ACID (VITAMIN B5)

Pantothenic acid deficiency severely inhibits antibody production, and this is exacerbated by a combined deficiency of vitamins B5 and B6.

ASCORBIC ACID (VITAMIN C)

Vitamin C is one of the anti-oxidant vitamins (along with Vitamin E, and Selenium) which is important as a de-toxifying agent in the removal of harmful allergic food substances, yeast metabolites and chemicals. Vitamin C tidies up each cell's chemistry after the ravages of an invading harmful chemical. Unused vitamin C cannot be stored in the body so must be taken in divided doses throughout the day.

VITAMIN E

The function of vitamin E in the body is similar to that of vitamin C, but vitamin E can be stored to some degree in the body, therefore it is unwise to take high doses.

VITAMIN A

Adequate vitamin A is essential for the maintenance of healthy skin and mucous membranes and aids in resisting invasion of those surfaces by Candida and other infectious organisms. It is essential for regeneration of a competent immune system. Vitamin A is stored in fatty tissues in the body and can be toxic in large doses so should only be taken under supervision.

ZINC

One of the most important minerals for maintaining healthy skin and mucous membranes and for wound healing and resistance to infection is zinc. It is also essential for maintaining the immune system.

MAGNESIUM, IRON, MANGANESE AND COPPER

These minerals are also essential for a competent immune system and iron deficiency is common amongst Candida sufferers. Copper deficiency is uncommon because it is a regular contaminant of our drinking water as a result of the use of copper piping.

FATTY ACIDS

Prostaglandins are chemicals manufactured by the body which control inflammatory reactions to toxins. Their production requires an adequate supply of the fatty acids gamma-linoleic acid and eicosapentaenoic acid which can be taken as a supplement to stimulate prostaglandin production. (These are available in Evening Primrose Oil).

Because of the possible toxicity of some vitamins and minerals when taken in excess, and because of the danger of a reaction to a non-active ingredient in a commercial supplement, it is advisable to seek the advice of a nutritionally oriented health professional.

CHAPTER 11

MOULD AVOIDANCE

Often, it is not enough to merely remove yeast and mould products from the diet, it may be necessary to reduce the exposure to mould spores from the atmosphere. When a mould cell matures, it releases millions of tiny spores into the atmosphere, relying on wind and air currents to distribute the spores far and wide. The spores are inhaled along with air and are trapped by the normal air cleaning mechanisms on the mucous membranes of the nasal and chest airways. The spores can immediately initiate a local allergic reaction such as an attack of asthma, or may be carried along with the mucus to the throat and then swallowed. Mould metabolites released by decaying mould spores in the gut can be absorbed into the bloodstream and carried to the brain or other organs where they may cause a toxic reaction.

The environmental conditions which encourage mould growth are dampness and darkness, so attempts to control mould growth are aimed at establishing more light and dryer conditions.

Mould very commonly occurs in:

Bathrooms which are poorly lit and poorly ventilated, particularly in the bath or shower area or in cupboards. Tile grouting, shower curtains, sliding shower screen tracks, damp and soiled towels and clothing are all sites which encourage mould growth.

Kitchens which have inadequate ventilation would be a source of environmental mould contamination especially in under-sink cupboards, in refrigerator door seals and in the water evaporating tray under self de-frosting refrigerators, on scored or worn wooden chopping boards.

Bedrooms contain bedding which can become damp from perspiration which may not dry out in poorly ventilated rooms and so encourage mould growth. Regular laundering and airing of bedding will minimize this risk.

Cupboards and store rooms where soiled or old clothing, shoes, leather goods, newspapers, books etc. are stored. Clothes which are damp or have been worn and put away without laundering will quickly become mouldy while laundered clothing will keep well in a cupboard.

Damp under-house areas, cellars or sheds (especially those with an earth floor) have a high mould level and should be avoided.

Carpeting collects dust and mould in the pile which is not removed by normal vacuuming techniques. Scatter rugs can similarly become soiled unless laundered frequently.

Old upholstered or overstuffed furniture or bedding contains mould which cannot easily be removed by cleaning.

Indoor plants have soil and moisture in the pot along with decaying organic matter which encourage mould growth.

Houses located in heavily timbered areas generally suffer from retained moisture which is not cleared because of shade and poor air circulation.

Decaying vegetable matter such as leaves and lawn clippings are very mouldy and mowing or raking will disturb millions of spores.

Fruits or vegetables stored in cupboards, pantry or sheds will quickly establish moulds, especially root vegetables such as carrots and potatoes.

It may not be possible to remove or clean up all sources of mould exposure, but, any improvement in the environment will certainly reduce the overall allergenic load and hopefully lead to an improvement and reduction of symptoms.

CHAPTER 12

EXERCISE
AND ATTITUDE

There are two factors which can greatly influence the outcome of a disease condition that do not involve avoidance of a favourite food. Vigorous physical exercise stimulates the production of chemicals in the body called endorphins, which have an action on the brain not unlike that of opium in that they reduce perception of pain and discomfort. For excercise to be an effective therapeutic tool, it needs to be performed at least once a day and is preferable if it is an exercise which you enjoy. It is advisable to obtain some help from a professional when designing an exercise program.

Laughter is another powerful stimulant to the production of endorphins, so one should *seek* out a happy, healthy environment in which to enjoy a sense of wellbeing. It is very easy to fall in the trap of becoming totally involved with one's own discomforts and to surround oneself with negative thoughts. Therefore, it is necessary, as with any disease, to shake off the negativism and to do some positive thinking. If you cannot help yourself on some occasions and have a "binge" on some detrimental food then it is necessary to avoid compounding the discomfort of the food reaction with a feeling of guilt. If it happens, enjoy it, and think about some positive way that the situation may be avoided in the future.

By combining the right amounts of all the measures mentioned in this book then there is a very good chance that you will be able to demonstrate that CANDIDA CAN BE BEATEN!

For those of you who wish to study the subject in greater detail, or are still confused by it all, we recommend these books:

The Missing Diagnosis by Dr C. Orion Truss, C. Orion Truss, 1983

The Yeast Connection by Dr William G. Crook, Professional Books, 1983

Food Intolerance by Robert Buist, PhD., Harper & Row, 1984

INDEX